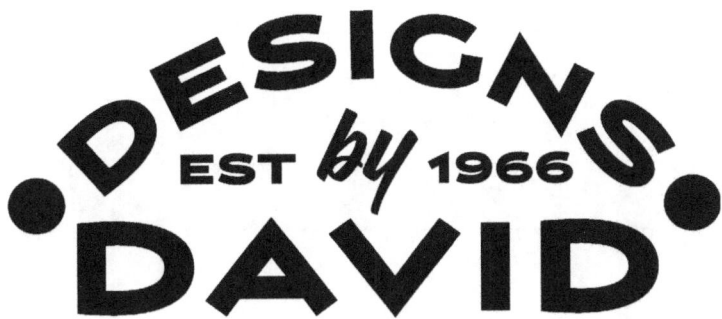

Faith Over Fear Journal

Copyright 2019 Designs By David all rights reserved. Reproduction or retransmission of these materials, in whole or in part, in any manner, without the prior written consent of the copyright holder, is a violation of copyright laws

www.ingramcontent.com/pod-product-compliance
Lightning Source LLC
Chambersburg PA
CBHW072152170526
45158CB00004BA/1610